YOU ARE HAPPINESS

How to Return to the Joy, Peace, and Love Already Within You

G. Tyler Wright

TranscendentWritings.com

ISBN-13: 9781234567890
ISBN-10: 1477123456

Cover design by: Art Painter
Library of Congress Control Number: 2018675309
Printed in the United States of America

CONTENTS

FOREWORD

Being full of joy and bliss is natural for everyone. Living as if this isn't true also seems to be natural for most people, but it isn't. It's taught by society, and anything that can be learned can be unlearned. A bad habit can be changed into a good one simply by replacing faulty understanding with correct knowledge.

If you are ready to connect to the part of you that is one with joy and peace, and live happier than ever before, then what are we waiting for! Let's begin our amazing journey to a new, bliss-filled experience of life!

1) THE NATURAL CHILD

As children, we are naturally full of joy. We laugh easily and smile for no reason. Love and delight shine through our eyes, and we play as if there were no other purpose to life. Everything is new, everything is fun, and life is lived in each fresh, exciting moment.

That joy is not something we achieved. It is what we are, before anyone teaches us to be anything else. For the first three or four years of life — with no instruction, no classes, no effort at all — we express it most of the day, every day.

And then, slowly, we learn to cover it up.

It isn't anyone's fault, and it isn't a conspiracy. It is simply what growing up in a structured world tends to do. We are taught to sit still, to wait our turn, to be quiet, to raise a hand before we speak, to save our enthusiasm for an appropriate time — which, it turns out, is almost never. Much of this is even necessary. But drip by drip, year after year, a quiet message sinks in: your spontaneous joy is a problem to be managed.

By the time we are grown, we have practiced that lesson so thoroughly that no one needs to enforce it anymore. We enforce it on ourselves. We walk past people without smiling. We sit for hours without once checking in with our own happiness. We trade play for productivity and call it maturity. The exuberant four-year-old is still in there — but we have spent years learning to keep her quiet.

Here is the proof of how strong that original joy really is: it took years of steady conditioning to dim it. If we weren't joyful at the core, it wouldn't have taken so long to disconnect us — and we wouldn't still, all these years later, ache to feel it again.

And we do ache for it. The longing never goes away; we just learn to reach for it in the wrong places — a drink to loosen up, a substance to feel free, a vacation to finally exhale. For a few hours the old joy breaks through, and we remember what it felt like simply to be alive. Then the inhibition closes back over it, and we go looking for the next escape. A surprising amount of what we call addiction is really just this: a buried joy, reaching for any door it can find.

But here is the good news, and it is the foundation of this entire book: the joy was never rooted out. It was only covered over. Anything that can be learned can be unlearned. A habit of disconnection can be replaced by a habit of connection. You do not have to manufacture happiness, or earn it, or chase it across the world. You only have to clear away what has been laid on top of it — and come home to what you already are.

That is what the rest of these pages are for. Not to give you happiness — you already have it. To help you remember the way back.

So let's begin.

2) PREPARING THE WAY

Experiencing our true inner bliss is the easiest, most natural activity in the world. We did this as children without taking one class or reading one book. Without any knowledge at all of what we were doing, day in and day out, for the first three or four years of our lives we expressed our bliss most of the day every day.

It took at least fourteen years of school to obliterate our connection to how to be, so we can see how strong our connection to our true inner spirit of joy was. If we weren't full of joy and bliss at our core, it wouldn't take so many years to disconnect us from ourselves. After all these years of programming, we wouldn't still need to connect with that bliss, and we wouldn't seek it through chemical means.

We need to become very clear about this truth. As long as we consider joy and happiness to be something outside of our truest nature, we won't accept it as our right. As long as we hold onto the structure of our programming, we will never tear down the walls that keep us from experiencing ourselves naturally and without shame.

Society is a big creation of humankind. No one person made it, but millions contributed to its foundations and billions of us sustain it every day. Each moment we spend silent, frowning, wrapped up in our worries about a future moment, instead of smiling or laughing and enjoying the moment we are experiencing, we are adding to the structure that is our current society. Every day which we fill more with work than with happiness is a day where we build our little section of an oppressive, soul-sapping society stronger and more unbreakable.

Many of us see the problem, but few realize how we willingly contribute to its continuation. When we perform the simple act of walking past someone without smiling or acknowledging their existence, we are expressing the teachings of society. When we sit at our desk for an hour or two without connecting with our inner joy, we are adding fuel to the engine of society. When we go to a job we hate, day after day, because we "have to", we sustain the very world we should be destroying.

Every time we find ourselves behaving in ways that we wouldn't when we were four, we have the very real possibility of acting through the teachings we have ingrained. When we choose order over fun, we are disconnecting from our inner bliss. When we accept a life full of work instead of play, we are expressing what our schools have taught us, not what our hearts yearn to experience.

It is imperative that we recognize where we really are, how deep down the rabbit hole of society we have gone in order to see that we must change. As long as we believe things aren't so bad - a couple of cups of coffee in the morning, a smoke or three during the day, a couple of beers in the evening aren't signs of the end of the world, right- we won't take any action to live life differently. We must begin to see that the world we are creating every day is not a world in which we can really be alive.

You create the world you live in. No one else lives in your same world. If you think this isn't true, sit down and talk with anyone about five different beliefs about the world. Talk about religion, politics, sex, or race and see if you live in their world. The beliefs you hold true shape the manner in which you experience your world in every moment.

If we believe God is watching and judging us, our world will be different from someone who believes their God lives within. If we believe the world is a place where everyone is out for themselves, our world is very different from someone who believes the world is a place that we all share, and that we must care for those who can't care for themselves. If we believe money makes the man, we live in a different world from someone who believes our value comes from our shared love and humanity.

When we understand the power we have – we create

and inhabit new worlds every day! – we can begin to consciously use our power to create a world more in the image of the joyful three-year-old we were, and less trapped in the programming of the adult we battle being. Then we can live in a world that looks more like what we would create if we knew we were creating a world.

A world that is in tune with our true nature includes more laughter, more love, more daily joy, a sense of belonging shared by all and an allowing for all to freely and shamelessly express the inner bliss that bubbles below the surface of life in every moment. This is a world full of smiling people who genuinely care for and about one another, not just for a small family, a select church family, or an insular clique of friends. This is a world where people care for people, regardless of color, nationality, or any of the many other boxes people are currently labeled with. It is also a world where we are all involved in activities that we enjoy and resonate with. We all follow activities we are passionate about. We live with an enthusiasm for life that raises the level of joy in the world everyday.

So how do we get to this point where we are creating worlds we really want to live in?

Once we understand how the world we currently see is a result of past beliefs held by each person, slightly different but fairly complementary beliefs, we can see that each individual has the power to agree or disagree every day to living in the present world. When we agree, we continue to keep our heads down and walk past people as if they don't exist. When we disagree, we look up and we smile. When we disagree, we make eye contact. We laugh and enjoy being alive. We awaken that four-year-old we have been taught all of our lives to subdue. We let many of the ways of the child come alive again.

When we start doing this, we find joy beginning to pervade our everyday life. We find our connection to our true bliss within becoming stronger and our expression of it more natural. We find ourselves living as we were intended to live.

We also find the need to add strange chemicals to our bodies is gone. When we are in tune with our inner bliss, we do not need alcohol or drugs anymore. Our healthy bodies produce all the joyful chemicals we need in just the right combination to have the experience of enjoying life now.

3) DIGGING OUT OF THE HOLE

Now that we understand where we really live, and how we got here, we can begin to make the changes necessary to begin living in a place we want to live. The changes we must make are small, but they combine to bring our lives into alignment with our inner nature. We've spent many years learning how to not be ourselves, and we will need to spend an equal amount of energy to undo these lessons and return to our true selves.

The good news is while we were fighting a daily battle as children when the lessons of school were obliterating our connections to ourselves, now we are reawakening these natural connections, so we are now going with nature instead of against it. Basically, we were going the wrong way, paddling upstream against a strong current, and now we will be rowing downstream with the flow, in the right direction.

We will reach our goal of daily happiness, joy and bliss in our lives in very little time. We will do this because it is our inner nature to do this. We've been trained to forget, but remembering yourself isn't really so hard once we understand that's what we're doing.

The most important step is the first one, and all it is is breathing. Become aware and breath in and out. You say, "I do this all the time, everyday already. I wouldn't be alive if I didn't!

This is true, but becoming aware means breathing in a conscious manner. Inhale deeply, exhale deeply. Do this now and feel the peace it brings. Deep inhalation, deep exhalation. Nothing could be simpler than this, right? So why do we forget this most basic of all actions when we need it the most? When we become stressed out about something or when we are in a difficult emotional situation, invariably we breathe in short shallow breaths. We don't realize it, but short breaths actually assist in maintaining a stressful physiology.

Deep breaths break us out of it. They allow the body to have more oxygen, which gets all the blood and the chemicals flowing better, which allows us to make better decisions and deal with things from a fuller perspective. Breathing also allows us to step back from the movement of a particular situation and see it from a more peaceful position. It basically takes us out of looking outward and moves us to a place of looking inward. And this inward vantage-point is a space of understanding, peace and solutions.

So learn to breath, learn to accept that the most basic action our body performs, when connected to consciously, is the single biggest gift our body has for our peaceful and joyous state of mind.

As small children we naturally run and laugh and play and breathe deeply. All of our activity demands we breathe deeply even if we aren't aware of it. When we argue, our breath becomes shallow. When we cry, we barely breathe and must gasp for breath. When we calm down, again we are breathing more broadly, and when we are again active and running, moments later we have deep happy breaths again.

So what was unconsciously natural for us as children must be consciously understood and practiced as an adult. Take time and breathe. Practice sitting and just breathing deeply. Focus all your energy on feeling the breath come in and go out of your lungs. Notice how the air feels cool coming in and warmer going out. Feel your chest expanding and contracting. Get familiar with your breath and recognize that when you need it, it is there for you.

When you feel yourself contracting, when you feel yourself in a space where you perceive problems and are anxious, you will realize that this is a time when you are focused on problems and are not breathing well. Learn how to recognize these moments and to consciously breathe deeply instead.

Many of us unconsciously already know the power of this action and use a prop to help us do this act many times a day. We take breaks with our breathing tool and we take deep breaths to feel good. Society doesn't allow us to go outside and just breathe deeply without feeling strange, but when we hold our breathing prop in-between our fingers we lose the shame and feel we are breathing in a socially acceptable manner.

Yes, smoking a cigarette is at its essence nothing more than finding an excuse to immerse yourself in the joy of breathing for a few minutes. As forms of smoking without nicotine are becoming more common, we can truly see it is not the chemical intake that we yearn for as much as the stress-relieving act of consciously breathing deeply.

School never outlawed breathing, but it did outlaw the energizing activities kids do that keep them breathing deeply. "Stop running, don't yell, slow down!" are all ways that the level of energy we had as children was diminished, and the unconscious connection with deep breathing was severed.

Now we must reconnect with our body and breathe deep and long and feel the joy that this brings.

EXERCISE 1: BREATHE

Sit in a comfortable position in a place without distractions and become aware of your breathing. Close your eyes if it helps you to pull your attention inside to your breath. Watch yourself breathing normally, then gradually take control of your breath.

Breathe in deeply and feel the air rushing inside your body. See it going in and picture the life-giving oxygen being distributed by your lungs into your bloodstream and into the whole of your body. Hold the breath and allow all the oxygen to give its energy to you. Then let your breath out, again in a long exhalation, discarding the carbon dioxide that has been created in the life-exchange occurring in your lungs. Let go of all the waste air, then sit still and empty for a moment.

Again, breathe in deeply, long and slow, filling your lungs as deeply as possible. Each time you do this you are helping to build your lung's capacity to retain and process more oxygen - basically improving your health. Sit and hold the air and allow the exchange to take place in your lungs. Exhale deeply and eliminate all the used breath that no longer has value to your body. Sit still again, completely empty, then repeat.

This time add a slow count, to five or seven or ten, whatever is most comfortable, and fully inhale. Hold your breath in for the same count, then exhale, again for the same count, and again hold empty for the same count. Move into a natural rhythm of breathing with your natural count, filling your lungs completely and emptying them totally again and again. Inhale: one, two, three, four, five. Hold full: one, two, three, four, five. Exhale: one, two, three, four, five. Hold empty: one, two, three, four, five. Keep your energy focused on breathing, and when you find a natural comfortable, deep rhythm, stay in it and continue with it. Don't let the thoughts of your day intrude on this time you are spending with your breath, but just breathe.

Set aside about ten minutes everyday to become re-acquainted with your deep breathing and you will soon see that it will become your friend whenever you need it during the day. Feel free to take this practice beyond your quiet space. Close your eyes and breathe for a few minutes at your desk or in a chair or anyplace you want during your day.

Once you have become comfortable with this breathing exercise, you'll find you're able to focus on your breath anywhere you are, however busy a place may be. This is when you'll be able to see that you've mastered your breathing and can call on its soothing properties whenever and wherever you need them to connect you to peace within.

4) ALLOWING SPACE

The next step in returning naturally to inner peace and joy is allowing space to exist in our mind. One huge difference between an adult and a child is the adult worries about almost every future event imaginable in life while the child's only preoccupation is with playing. In the morning, we worry about how we look, what clothes we should wear, how we smell, how clean our teeth are, what time it is, will I be late. Then we leave the house and a new set of worries appear. We worry about traffic when we drive, and we worry about our car when traffic doesn't take all of our attention. We worry about finding a good parking space, we worry about clocking in or arriving on time. All of these same worries fill our minds at least five mornings a week. The same thoughts, replayed day after day, week after week, month after month, and year after year after year after year ad infinitum.

Whatever our situation during the day, we have thoughts and worries to accompany them. When working we worry about the speed and the accuracy of our work. When eating we worry about health, taste, and gaining weight, not necessarily in that order!

While these are examples of local thoughts - thinking and worrying related to a particular situation - we also have more global concerns, more standard worries to fall back on when local worries subside for a few minutes. When we are standing in a line, when we stop worrying about how long we will have to continue standing in line, if we don't hop onto our phones, we have a few free minutes where we can worry about money – or the lack thereof, love – or the lack thereof, sex -or the la -you get it! We worry about the state of our lives, health, relationships, children, friends, job, political situations.

Heaven forbid if our phone battery dies while we are standing in line. Then we have nothing to occupy us while we wait. So we look around and see everyone else on their phone, and we start to worry about what they are thinking if you aren't on your phone too. We worry about what others think about us, and if others like us. We worry about being good looking enough, normal enough, smart enough. We worry or fear that we are lacking some key element and that the world will expose us for the fraud that we really are!

There are so many things to worry about that we do not have a moment of stillness. We have become so used to thinking about all the things going on in life that we find even the thought of not thinking about something in every waking moment strange or unnatural.

As a child we wondered when we could play, what we could play, then we played. When we played, we didn't worry about things beyond playing. We didn't even worry about the next game. We played and enjoyed where we were at and what we were doing.

Complications only started when we had been indoctrinated enough to disconnect with the joy in the activities of the present moment. When we were forced to do actions we didn't want to do or didn't care about, our minds began to wander and the unhealthy habit of worrying and thinking too much was born.

Have you ever stopped to not think for a minute? Yes, to *not* think. Sadly, too few of us have thought about not thinking. Now that's an irony! One of the most important thoughts to occupy our minds with is about not occupying our minds with thoughts at all! Doing this is the gateway to returning to the joy we experienced in childhood, before we became so addicted to thinking that we forgot about being.

For the few who have thought about not thinking, and have even tried to do it, we are a minority of the population. Those who have succeeded even for two minutes are far fewer. We live so much in the thoughts and worries of the mind that to turn it off appears not to be an option. Why would we want to stop it, the thought goes. After all, we are our thoughts, right? We live inside the mind, we believe we are the mind, or that it is ours, and that when it thinks, it is important to listen.

Far too few of us have ever thought about stepping outside the chatter of thought for a few minutes to see what life is like on the other side. We think it is natural to think, and in fact that thinking can't stop. "I think, therefore I am," is Descartes' famous quote. A few minutes of peace and quiet, without the incessant thinking mind can show you that this isn't remotely true. A few silent minutes with a quiet mind can change your life.

As children, we were much more carefree and thought free. Yes, we did think, but no, at an early age we were not addicted to thinking like we are now. For many of us thinking has no connection to the joy in our lives. Only in the moments when thought has subsided are we able to feel happiness welling up from within. Then we think, and the happiness fades. While thought can be a trigger to experience joy, most often incessant thought does just the opposite.

So how do we break out of this addiction that keeps us separated from our bliss? The answer is the same one that you have already learned: by breathing consciously. When we understand how we are really arranged within, then we can see how and why this is the answer.

Our mind is a tool made for thinking, nothing more, nothing less. It is rightly used to consider a situation, and when the consideration is finished, it should be silent. We experience the mind talking because we have what can be called focused awareness or attention which we continually give to one thing or another. Using awareness, we understand that we are the watcher of the mind, not the actual activity of thinking.

If we don't realize we have or we are attention that can focus on whatever it wants, we find ourselves like a dog, entranced by the moving ball, or in our case, the moving thoughts of the mind. Movement grabs our attention and holds it, but that doesn't mean whatever we are watching is what we are. When the mind moves, we have the choice to watch it or not. Very few people ever realize this simple fact.

Every thought is not us, and every thought is not so important that it has to be watched. When we realize that we are much more intimately the attention we give to our thoughts and not the thoughts themselves, then we can begin to control where this attention goes. We need to see that this experience of life we have goes through the choices we make with our attention, and most importantly we are the master of this choice.

So, when the mind begins worrying about something, we can choose to watch it and identify with the thoughts as our own, or we can choose to let it think, and watch something else. There is another show on the tv, another channel to turn to. Instead of the words of the mind, turn to the feeling of the breath.

When we watch our breathing instead of our thoughts, we can see that the feeling of breathing is enough motion to attract our attention. We see that there is enough substance in the structure of the breath to keep our attention entertained. We find that attention on the breath allows our inner joy to arise.

We also see that thinking will not survive too long without the energy it receives from attention. At times thinking is nothing more than a dancing child, moving back and forth seeking mommy's attention. And when mommy doesn't look, after awhile the child stops dancing around trying to get attention. The creative child will stop one movement and come up with something more interesting to try and get mommy's attention, and the mind is nothing if not a creative child. When it sees the average thoughts don't draw attention, it comes up with amazing, extraordinary thoughts to make us look. Ideas to change the world, understandings to enlighten the masses, thoughts to transform our life all pop up when the mind becomes desperate for attention. If we are able to continue focusing on our breathing instead of on the great thoughts – yes labelled great by the thinking mind! – then we will really begin to take control of our experience of life, and our connection with our inner joy.

EXERCISE 2: ATTENTION

Sit in your quiet space and practice your breathing as in Exercise 1. Consciously experience the four parts of the breathing cycle. Each breath begins with the inhalation. Put your full attention on this action. Feel the air as it comes in. Be aware that thought likes most to begin with the inhalation and allow your attention to full embrace the experience of the breath coming in instead. You may feel a tingling sensation with the in-breath starting in the lungs and expanding to your whole body. Allow it to sweep like a wave through you and enjoy it. Next, on the in-pause, sit in the silence that is the experience of full lungs. Feel the peace of this stillness and silence and allow the waves of the thrill of breathing to wash over you. Let the sounds you may hear become your mind, watching them as they arise and subside, not attached to them, just hearing them, then returning attention to the silence within. By this time, if it has not happened naturally, move your attention to the space of your lungs or heart and out of your head.

Next allow the breath to go out. Feel the rush of the air and enjoy the sensation of release. Enjoy the freedom of letting go of everything as the breath leaves. The mind has no place in this release, and usually does not try to steal you away at this point in the cycle. Feel the push of the last of the air as it leaves your body, then rest again in the stillness that arrives with the empty lungs. Rest in this space as before, and dive into the feeling of emptiness. Dive deeper still and see that there is nothing in the emptiness but your joy, just waiting for you to experience it.

Repeat the cycle and go even deeper into the feelings of the breath as it comes in, as it rests inside, and as it leaves, keeping the attention on the silence and emptiness and stillness the receding breath creates. The mind may try to steal your attention away from your inner peace, but when you become aware of this theft, simply return your awareness to your breath and your space within your chest. Breathe in, hold, breathe out, hold and feel the peace of this experience again and again.

Ten minutes a day spent focusing on the breath will allow you to learn control of your attention. It will show you your intimate connection to attention, and teach you that you are not your mind, but that the mind - just like the body - is a tool to use to experience and enjoy life in this world.

5) ADDICTED TO MIND

Starting from the earliest moments of childhood, we watch the mind doing its thing. We see the mind interacting first with the world, then later with its memories of the world. The mind is made of thoughts, and these thoughts have been our constant companion. As a young child the mind was used to name and understand the world around us. The things around us became objects with names and functions, and we used the mind to understand them. One of the functions of the mind, memory, was very useful in helping us to learn about the world around us. One of the first things we learned was we enjoyed having fun, and the mind assisted us in having fun by identifying things that were fun, remembering these activities, and staying out of the way to allow us to experience the joy of doing inherent in the experience.

As we became older, thinking continued to assist us, but it also started to rebel. When we found that we could not do only the things we enjoyed, it expressed its dislike for the lack of control by wishing it was somewhere else, and by labelling the current situation bad. At this moment, the mind learned to think as an experience was happening instead of getting out of the way. It also learned to wish for a reality beyond what was currently happening. It found this method of escaping from the present moment was a viable option to living through a less than desirable experience.

In grade school these tendencies were reinforced by more and more situations for the mind to rebel against. Instead of being a tool with which to experience and enjoy the world, the mind became a filter for the world. It was always on, always thinking, and never saw a time when it should stop. It created a reality that always went through what it thought. If we believed one thing to be good and another to be bad, it shaded reality accordingly. It decided candy was good and apples were bad, and created an affinity for candy and an aversion towards apples. Getting dirty was fun, taking a bath wasn't, and it reacted accordingly with complaints and fussing when bath time arrived.

The mind formed a set of beliefs about everything it encountered and everything it was taught, and in doing so, it created a new world to live in. It provided an additional service to us in the form of a judge. Everything we encountered it judged as good or bad. Things, people, situations, everything was graded and classified and put in a box so that the next time we encountered it, we would know how we should react to it. For each of us our mind created our own personal reaction to literally everything that happened. It used memory to make sure that it reacted the same way each time to the same stimulus. The mind made sure to be consistent to the person it saw itself as being in each experience of life. Never could it enjoy a bath if its past experiences said baths were awful. Never could it like an apple, if only candy tasted good.

As adults we don't realize that our relationship with the mind was ever any different. We don't remember it was once a useful tool until it became part of its creation of a person. Now we are addicted to watching it think, and we are ignorant of the fact that its thinking is something we are watching, not something we create. The mind thinks, attention watches, and the seam between the two in minimized and goes unquestioned.

It's only when we sit still and watch our breath that we create a situation where we can begin to see the true nature of the mind. When we are able to stop the flow of thinking for a moment, we can see that we are looking at the mind think instead of falling for its unexamined belief that it is just us thinking.

With this simple observation and the accompanying understanding, we can begin to return to the place where we were early in life, when the mind was a tool that could navigate the world, then get out of the way when we were inside an experience.

When we delve deeply into the experience of con-sciously breathing, we see that each cycle is full of experience. An act as simple as breathing is usually so mechanical as to be ignored, but in reality it is full of activity to be enjoyed when the mind gets out of the way. Each cycle brings fresh bliss bubbling up from inside, when we pay intimate attention to each component of the cycle. If such a simple action as inhaling and exhaling can be so full of joy, imagine what we are missing by thinking throughout other activities instead of letting the mind subside and al-lowing attention to experience life anew.

Thinking as most of us do it is nothing but an ad-diction to experiencing a mind-made world instead of living in this reality of ever-new sensations and experiences.

In reality nothing we do has been done before, but we never take the time to realize this. The attention that you command today has the experience stored in memory of a whole day that the attention you commanded yesterday didn't. We change and grow everyday, every moment, and all that we see and do is colored by the growth we always experience. When we stop and see that life is always new, like we knew instinctively as a child, then we can begin to allow the mind to subside when we are living, and to assist in activities as needed instead of filtering every moment of life.

6) MIND VERSUS EMOTION

Another experience that our mind controls is our emotions. Many of us are unaware of this connection. We think emotions just arise, but the truth is that emotions are triggered by the mind. However the mind interprets an event dictates how the body responds. This response from the body is the emotion. Once the mind has labelled something good or bad, it ties feelings of happiness or sadness or anger into the experience. When the mind decides all apples tastes bad, the label it creates comes with all the feelings that it associates with bad things.

When we feel angry at someone or something, the feeling starts from the mind's interpretation of an event. If someone says, "You look bad," and we interpret this as a statement mocking our appearance, we can feel upset. When we replay the statement, we can go deeper and deeper into the range of negative feeling emotions. We can become angry, we can go deeper and become livid, as we add negative thoughts to the statement. If the person then says,

"No, I meant the good bad, not the bad bad," our whole demeanor can change in an instant. The mind interprets the words as good and the anger is gone. Instead happiness arises as we now feel the effect of the mind accepting a compliment. We can feel joyous as we go deeper into the experience of positive words.

Thoughts are the trigger for all emotions, but they call up the range of emotions in different ways. In order to feel negative emotions like sadness, anger, fear, and pain the mind must take an active role in creating a picture and sustaining the image in order to feel the feeling. If while we are in a negative emotion we can look at how we are doing it, we will see that we are actively thinking, over and over, about how bad something is.

We can also ask a child when they are in one of these emotions, "How are you able to stay sad?" Many children will be able to tell a story of what they are running through their mind or describe a picture of what they are seeing. Adults use the same mental process to create and sustain these emotions.

When it comes to positive emotions like happiness, joy, peace, contentment, and bliss our minds behave differently. While there is still a triggering statement or image, the mind does not have to work as hard to activate or to sustain the emotion. The mind can work as hard, but only when it is getting in the way of experiencing the emotion. When the mind is able to get out of the way of the experience of the emotion, the positive feeling can flow forth freely and easily.

The difference is like that between swimming upstream and downstream. When we're in the negative emotions, we're swimming upstream, against the flow, and against our true nature. When we are in a positive emotion, we're going with the current, and we're allowing our true nature to shine forth. The mind only has to turn in the positive direction, and our inner nature will do the rest. As long as the mind can let go and stay out of the way, we'll continue in the good feeling emotion. When the mind cannot let go, that's when it must work harder to sustain the emotion. Like throwing a ball, when we can fling our arm and release the ball, it can fly through the air. When we fling our arm and then don't let go of the ball, we must run with the ball in order for it to travel anywhere.

 Mind is intimately attached to emotion, and useful in achieving any emotional experience we desire. Since this is the case, then why don't we all use it to our benefit? If you could dial up any emotion you wanted, would you choose to be sad all day, or happy? Happy of course! So why aren't all of us happy all day every day? And when we get tired of being happy, we can dial it up a notch and feel blissful or dial it back a little into peace or contentment.

Now that we know the choice is ours, we can certainly decide, right now, to choose happiness much more often.

What is the best and easiest way the mind triggers happiness? Through thoughts of gratitude. When we can think of the things we are grateful for, we immediately trigger happiness in our body. We can ask ourselves "What am I grateful for?" and watch a list develop right before our mind. Dwelling on these things during the day makes for a transformed life.

We are grateful for our loved ones, our spouse, our children, parents, friends, family. We are grateful for our safety and comfort, our jobs or businesses that provide us with the things we need and enjoy having. We are grateful for our environment, our country, our world, and even our universe, all of which allow us to experience life. We are grateful for life itself, for that which created us, for the essence that we experience as ourselves. We could even be grateful for the fact that we can experience gratitude and that it leads to happiness, and for being able to experience happiness. We can be grateful for our breath, for our connection with the stillness, for our ability to delve into the silent peace between each breath.

The list is truly endless if we begin to ask, then allow the answers to flow in.

When we find the thoughts that resonate best with us and bring the most happiness, we can then experience the happiness, joy, or peace that thinking about them opens us to experiencing. Let the mind hold the ball (think the thought) then throw the ball (let go of the thought) and feel the ball flying through the air (experience the emotion).

As simple as throwing a ball, we can take control of our emotional states and feel positive emotions whenever we want to. Even when we find the mind dwelling on things that make the body experience negative emotions, it is our choice whether to continue with the chain of thought the mind has, or to move to a better one. We can zoom in and focus on any negative detail or experience, or we can zoom out to the wonderful life that supports it all and appreciate the whole. Yes, a moment may be full of negative or challenging situations, and yes, we have the choice to decide how to interpret each and every one of them. We also have the choice to see things in the wider scope of life, and there can be something to appreciate when we choose to do so.

The anonymous driver can show us one of their fingers in a traffic jam, our boss can berate our work, our spouse can yell at us, and we can feel negative emotions with all of these experiences. But after the initial triggering, we can take control and deal with the situation from a space where we are not controlled by what others do, but by our own preferences. We can choose to thank the person in the other car for their feedback and be grateful that we only saw their finger! We can thank our boss for expressing his opinion -since it was probably worth exactly what we paid for it! We can thank our spouse for letting it out since communication, however given, is better than not communicating. We can come up with hundreds of other ways to see these situations, and to become happy with them, if we knew that this was an option, and if we exercised our options.

Now we know we have the choice, so it is just a matter of beginning to choose them and experience the positive emotions that go along with better choices. Just because someone else expects a certain reaction to their negative action doesn't mean we must behave as an automaton and give them their expected reaction! Why should we carelessly give away our power to circumstances perceived by others in a negative light? We are, of course receptive to constructive thoughts, but we are in control of how we receive and interpret input from others.

The society we live in teaches us to react to the emotion of another in kind with that same emotion. If some is angry, we are expected to react in anger in return. If someone shares kind words, we receive them happily and respond in that fashion. The truth is we can respond however we choose. We do not have to live over half of our lives on the dark side! We can decide to live in positive emotions, and then do it. When someone tries to pull us into their moment of drama, we are not obligated to go. We can say no thank you to their offer, and continue to enjoy the peace or the happiness or the joy that we are in.

What goal can be achieved by joining someone else in negativity? Is the goal more important than our state of joy? If we can ask ourselves these simple questions instead of unconsciously reacting to a negative stimulus, we will find that the answer most of the time will allow us to stay in our joy.

Yes, of course there are times when we need to be stern, strict, forceful etc., but that doesn't mean that we lose our connection with the inner flow of joyful emotions. We can bring forth the persona as needed in a given situation, and at the same time we can still feel the inner serenity that we know never vanishes when we keep it in our attention.

7) A PHYSICAL REMINDER

While the mind can drive the body to experience a variety of emotions on command, the body can remember emotions and tie them to a certain gesture or movement. The most common example of this is a smile. When we smile we feel joyful emotions inside. A smile is an action the mind has connected with good feelings, and it acts as a trigger to bring up positive feelings whenever it arrives. If we realize we have a built-in system of making ourselves feel good whenever we want to, will we now use it more often? When the body smiles, happy emotions are experienced. The mind has no choice but to subside and allow positive feelings to flow.

When others smile, we respond in kind. A smile is a universal experience of happiness. When we share it, others are happy too. A smile is like the fire on the end of a candle. When we share it, we are lighting the candle of those with whom we have shared it. Not a fake smile either, as we can all tell when someone has moved their lips to mimic a smile. A real smile involves the mouth, the cheeks, the eyes – really the whole face. So when we share a genuine smile, we not only feel it inside, but we light up the world around us as well. In many moments in life, there is no greater gift to give ourselves and others than a smile.

The smiling habit reminds us to connect to our inner joy on a regular basis. It allows us to align with our inner nature and be joyful in the moments of our lives. In our moments alone, a smile should be our companion. Thoughts of wellbeing follow, and life has a light that harkens back to childhood where a smile was easy and often felt.

you appreciate the challenging moments or the moments of adversity because they allow you to savor the moments of joy even more. Let them experience someone who can appreciate a larger perspective of life beyond the momentary irritations. Maybe, just maybe, your smile will introduce the other person to their smile as well!

8) UNDERSTANDING FOCUSED ATTENTION

Attention is the means by which we experience the world. If something doesn't demand our attention, it is not part of our world. When it does get our attention, it exists to us.

When we move from one room to another and close the door between the two, the first room becomes nothing more than a memory and an assumption. We assume it still exists as we remember it, and since most times this is true, we feel secure in believing it is part of our world. In reality our world is really only what is in front of us at the moment. The room we are in has the chance to have our attention; the one we left does not. But our attention isn't even on the entire room we currently inhabit, but on the tiny section that we are dealing with.

Our vision has a focal point and the rest is the periphery of our focus. That is really all we are able to put varying degrees of attention on at any one time. A point of primary attention and a background make up our world at any one time. The assumptions of the mind through memory fill in the gaps to make us believe we have a larger picture at any given moment.

The mind doesn't have two trains of thought moving forward simultaneously. It can only think one thought at a time. We may be thinking of two separate things, but each is thought of individually, and alternatively when we may believe they are being thought of together.

Our attention is like a spotlight, able to go to one thing, then another. The fun part is that we can control where we put our attention at any time. For all intent and purpose, we *are* our attention. What we pay attention to creates our experience of life. This being the case, it is very important to understand this and to apply it to making our lives reflect what we want to experience.

The mind is not attention, but is guided by attention, not the other way around. We decide where to put attention, the mind follows and begins thinking about where attention has been placed. If we change our minds, we have moved attention somewhere else.

The mind can be like a dog on a leash, pulling us here and there at its whim, but we always need to remember who is holding the leash and who is being held by it. The mind can go off on a tangent, but attention can bring it back to its focus. Just like a dog owner who sees an open field and releases the leash to let the dog run wild for a while, we can let go of the mind to let it run for a while. The important understanding that too few of us have is that we are not controlled by the dog, but can call it back on the leash at any moment we choose.

We have the choice in every moment to watch or not to watch the thoughts running through our heads. Too few of us realize this, having instead identified ourselves as the thinking in the mind. The reality is the mind can think, and we can pay attention to something else. Try this now. Start to think about what clothes you want to wear tomorrow, then in the middle of this thought move your attention to the tree outside your window, or the nearby wall.

When we do this we see who is in control of thoughts, and we see what it is that gives energy to thinking: attention. Without attention, thought stops pretty quickly. Thought may try to start itself up again with a word or two, but if we do not pay attention, if we give the mind no energy, thought cannot go far.

The thing about attention, though, is that when we are unaware of its power, we let it roam without control. Instead of behaving as the master with the leash, we let attention behave as a dog who sees a butterfly. We chase the butterfly all around the park, following, jumping, trying to catch it and never succeeding. Only our butterfly is mental noise. Whatever moves holds our attention. Whatever new thought arises, even if it is the same one we thought yesterday, and the day before, and the day before, just because it is the pretty butterfly or the moving ball in front of our attention, it is what we will allow the mind to be occupied with, and it is where the attention will follow.

If we were to realize the nature of attention is to follow movement, we would begin to take back control from the inconsequential thoughts that fill the foreground of our days to the background of joy and bliss that is our inner nature. We would begin to understand that we could stay as connected with our joy as we choose, understanding that the only time we move away from it is when we allow attention to follow the mind instead of staying with the awareness of our true inner happiness.

Until we know we have a choice, we usually don't change. If we are in a restaurant where we see everyone else ordering orange juice, we may always do the same and order orange juice, but we may be surprised to find out that they also sell mango juice, apple juice and cranberry juice.

Our relationship with the mind is the same. We think we are the mind, or we think that we must follow the direction of its thoughts, until one day we can be surprised to find out that we are not our thoughts. We are not the slave to their whims.

What we are is the watcher of our thoughts. We are the attention that powers and guides thoughts to go where we choose.

EXERCISE 4: MOVING ATTENTION TO HAPPINESS

A great way to really experience what we have just learned is to watch our minds in action. Sit in a comfortable, quiet place and start to think. Just start thinking about anything you want. Think about your day, or yesterday, and just let the mind flow freely.

As you do this, watch the thoughts as they occur. Be conscious of each movement as the thought train begins to leave the station. Watch the mind as it moves from one place to another. Be aware of how you may have started to think about the flowers in your garden and are now thinking about your best friend's wedding. Be aware of how the train moved from one subject to another to another to another. Allow it to flow, but don't become totally lost in its movement.

Now just as your mind is in the middle of a great exploration of why this or how that happened, remove attention from the train of thought and place it on the wall nearby or in front of you. Feel as if you have moved the center of your awareness outside of yourself and over to the wall. Stay with your focused attention on the wall for several minutes, or for as long as you can. Focus on feeling the wall, on becoming one with the wall.

As you do this, thinking has no energy. You have taken the supply of power away from thought and placed it on attention instead.

Next move your attention into your chest. Feel the space within your body and keep your attention there. You can close your eyes if it helps you focus better. You can also move the center of your attention just a little, just a few inches to the left or right every few minutes to allow you to stay focused on the space in your chest.

Attention likes movement, so if you move it a little bit, it is still able to get the sensation of movement, instead of needing to watch the mind move.

Now as you sit in the feeling inside your chest, begin to be aware of the background of it all, of the peace and stillness that has always been there, in the periphery, but not in the center of your attention. Bring the focus of your attention onto this peace, and feel it expanding. Feel yourself going deeper into it and experience the various flavors it has to offer. As you go deeper, feel the energy of peace growing into happiness. Enjoy the happiness and the joyous feeling, then go deeper into this and feel the bubbles of bliss.

Stay with the feeling of your inner nature and recognize this as your true core and essence. All of this is within, just waiting to be experienced. It should be a very familiar place to you, because it is the same place you easily lived in and expressed from as a young child.

9) UNDERSTANDING MIND AND ATTENTION

The mind thinks. It plays with thoughts, putting words together, forming ideas, moving concepts around, making things fit into logical relationships. It puts ideas into boxes to better understand and relate one concept to another. It categorizes concepts, creating hierarchies of importance and of degree. It judges actions good and bad. It remembers events as it wants to - not necessarily as they were. It forms beliefs that essentially color the world in its own image and inform the new inputs to this world accordingly.

Mind is an essential tool for living in this world. Its primary purpose is to assist us in better navigating through this world. It does this by creating a worldview which it uses to understand how things work and to better react to changes and predict future actions. It is the reasoning aspect of mind that separates us from animals. The collective use of mind is what we can thank for the current societies in which we live.

Mind has actually taken its job to a level beyond which it was intended. In helping us to better navigate the world, and by creating individualized worlds to do this, it has taken us away from our inner nature. By creating a world that is so enthralling and always in need of stimulus classification, it has drawn our attention away from what is the most important thing of all.

Mind is a learned construct. We were not born knowing how to think as we do today. We did not know words but learned them as we grew. We did not know how to put actions and reactions together but learned this relationship as we grew. The same can be said of most of the functions of the mind. Thinking as we know it today used innate tools in a manner taught to us by our society and environment.

We can see the pliability of mind by recognizing that the minds of various people in different cultures around the world use mind in different ways to form a large variety of perspectives on how the world is and should be. Some people have minds that allow them to see a world where people should be treated as lessor human beings because of their sex, or their sexual preferences. Others have minds that allow them to believe some people should be regarded as lessor human beings because of their skin color, culture or religious beliefs. Some people use their minds to emphasize the differences between people, while others use their minds to see the similarities.

The glass is half empty to some and half full to others. The decisions mind makes drastically changes the world that each of us live in from that of another. When we understand all these choices mind has made for us that shape our worldview are arbitrary, we begin to see the truth of the world we believe we live in. We see the opinions we hold are not really that solid. We see the worldviews they create are easily changed. We see the world we believe we live in is not so real after all.

When we meet a person we have prejudged as belonging to a particular group, many of us may expect them to behave one way that conforms to our preconceived notions. Then when we get to know them and they are real people and not a stereotype, we can either change our opinion of the person and maybe even realize the generalizations we have assumed about others like them are possibly incorrect, or we can decide this person is an exception to a rule that is still true. Or we can believe we are being tricked by this person, and that they really are the way we believed them to be all along.

The direction mind chooses is determined by the belief structure it holds about itself, or about the type of person it thinks it is. If it holds the label of being right always, then it is harder to change. If it holds the label of being open to new things, it reacts in a different manner.

This shows that although we are all born with a mind, how it is trained and our subsequent usage of it are why the world it creates is different for each of us. Different input to mind as it is growing produces the myriad of different outputs of adult minds in the world.

The uses of these minds are as varied as there are people, from those who use it to survive day by day, finding food and shelter where they can, scraping by to make it through each day, to the mind that makes decisions and moves people and money around like pieces on a chess board, touching and changing the lives of millions every day with a decision. Billions of examples are in between these extremes.

Minds may start at similar places, but they end up dramatically different. No two are alike, not even two born and raised moments apart. Sometimes twins grow up and have very similar outlooks on life, and other times they are very different people. Siblings are the same. Some are close to one another and their worldviews fit together well, and others are like night and day. The mind can be surrounded by the same input possibilities, but the choice of which inputs to receive and ingrain determines the ultimate state of the mind. This is where the power of attention comes in.

Attention is the power of focus that we all have. Either it is pointed at something, and the mind sees it and reacts to it, or the attention ignores it and it does not exist to the mind. Every day most of the things our bodies are near are ignored. Our senses can only take in a limited amount of information in an extremely limited bandwidth of sight, sound, smell, taste and touch. Animals show us that our senses can be very limited compared to theirs, and instruments that can see beyond the wavelengths of light than we can, or ones that can hear much better than us also show the limitations of the human body to interpret the world around us. Even within the tiny spectrum in which our senses operate, we see one thing at a time when surrounded by millions of possible inputs.

When two babies sit side by side, one could be drawn to the picture in front of them on the wall, while the other could be drawn to the toy sitting in the corner of the room. Someone comes in and takes the toy, upsetting the second child, but being nearly oblivious to the first one, still intent on the picture. Meanwhile the other pictures on the other walls, the table with food and the bureau with a mirror on top do not exist for either baby yet, as their attention has not been drawn to them.

Our whole lives are the same, with some things drawing our attention and other things not. Many worlds of things pass us by every day, unnoticed. A change in what we notice offers the possibility of living in a very different world, guided both by attention and by how attention activates the mind to use the data it receives to create the world it lives in.

While we all turn out differently even though we start with tools that are nearly the same, almost all of us end up living in worlds that are compatible although not identical to each other. We intersect with others everyday who live in worlds that we barely recognize. If we could take a tour of someone else's world, we would find many strange things, some familiar thoughts, and a lot of things that are shifted ever so slightly to be aligned to the particular worldview being accepted.

Politically we can see this playing out in our daily lives. Some people use one media source to see a frightening world of terror, and others use another media outlet to see a world that doesn't care enough for the weak. Others still watch media that tells stories with a little of each of the others. Every outlet labels sections of the other outlet's output as untrue. The world we live in is shaped by the media we pay attention to.

The information that interests us, that grabs our attention, is what we process. The rest does not exist to us or is nothing more than ignorant background noise. In the age of information, we can see that people are getting further apart as they can now delve into the information that most interests the attention and there is now enough of this information to fill a day spent ingesting it.

As little as twenty years ago, information about the world mainly came to us through a few sources and was dispensed two or three times a day, absorbed by most of us once a day. Now we are inundated with this same information multiplied by a million or a billion. It is always available, always "on", telling us what is happening on all points of the globe. Others are always available to give us their interpretation of all of these events filtered through their individual or collectively shared worldview. If our attention is drawn to an occurrence in the world or a specific topic, the mind can truly follow it as deeply as it desires, all day long.

Our world has expanded to encompass the activity of so many strangers as to make the one person we are most intimately aware of seem inconsequential by comparison. There are sites and shows where we can watch the lives of others develop right before our eyes. There are sites we can go to and watch the highlights of the lives of our friends and acquaintances. So much activity always is happening for us to choose to watch. So many things occurring to continually draw us outside of ourselves, away from what is most important for us to be in tune with. Maybe we need a site that tells us to stop looking at all the sites, turn off the net and the other screens, and tune in to our inner world!

We can definitely agree that there are many flavors of entertainment in the world, and we love to be entertained. We pay more for entertainment than almost anything else. Entertainment is so prevalent that more than likely, we are leaving the age of information and entering the age of entertainment. Those who entertain us are some of the highest paid people in the world, so there is without a doubt a value to the act of entertainment in the world today. From silly to profound, from action packed to sublime, from observatory to participatory, entertainment comes in all shapes and sizes. The one thing that all entertainment has in common is that it is all a distraction from our thinking mind.

When we are truly entertained, we are completely engaged in the act in front of us. We are not thinking about what we should eat or worrying about what we will do tomorrow. We are in the moment of the action totally. We are lost in the movie or play, we are engulfed in the game. Whatever it is, our attention is fully involved, and our mind is being used as a tool to facilitate the experience.

Could it be that this is why entertainment is such a valuable commodity in the world today? We have become so addicted to thinking that we would pay an exorbitant amount of our money and time just to have something to distract the mind from its incessant thought for a short time. We don't know how to stop the mind ourselves, so we turn to the drug called entertainment, if not to the drug called alcohol or drugs, to bring us to ourselves, for a few moments during our day.

We need all of these distractions to make us feel

good, happy or at peace. We use all of these activities to take us to the space within, beyond all activity, to the space we lived in as young children, in touch with the joy inherent inside themselves, brought out by literally every action they do.

When we experience each of the acts of life as new and fresh, we need to place our attention on them, as opposed to thinking about an experience as rote and repeating a menial habit. When we can focus on living instead of running on autopilot, we can begin to see our lives are infinitely entertaining, and that the mind shouldn't be the one having all the fun. When we don't pay attention, the mind takes over and thinks through the very act of living.

Realize this: the mind has taken over life for many of us. We don't experience without thought inter-preting or interrupting or filtering or categorizing. We don't just live anymore. The mind always gets in-volved and says, "Oh I did this before," or "This is just like..." It turns the potentially joy-infused events of life into mundane occurrences not as worthy of our attention as just thinking through them is.

To a child, all things are new and unique and fun. They pay attention to their lives. They do not allow thought to move unchecked through the fabric of their days.

When we really learned to think, we started to get hooked on the importance of our opinions. We started to place activities in boxes that we totally understood. Once we understand something, we don't have to pay it attention any longer, so we can think through the doing the next time. More and more things fell into this classification or judgement with our developing minds. We didn't notice that each day thinking took over the tasks of our lives, we also lost touch with the joy of living inherent in paying attention to life. In effect the joy of thinking replaced the joy of life. Instead of connecting with the inner joy and happiness within us all, we connected with the sense of satisfaction thinking gives when the mind believes it understands something.

Attention and mind are not always a mix that creates discord and boredom. They do not necessarily lead to an existence needing distraction to cope. The way the societies of the world use it today leads down this path, but this doesn't have to be the only way.

We can instead take the power back from the mind and allow attention to go within more often. We can allow the mind to be one tool, but not the only tool and filter of life. We can take control of when we think and when we don't. Most importantly we can also control *what* we think about and what we don't. We are not the slaves to our mind, but its master.

By wielding the power of attention, we take back that control. When we set our priorities and stick to them, we begin to train the mind to follow attention where we want to go, instead of wherever the whims of thought carry us.

10) PRIORITIZE WHAT'S REALLY IMPORTANT

Prioritizing your state of mind is not something taught in school. Amazingly most churches do not major in this thought process either. Instead we are taught in society to prioritize making money. School teaches the primacy of order and an education in a specific discipline. Various churches teach various worldviews, and a few teach how to approach life.

If we look at why we do anything in life, we see that we do it for the state of mind that it triggers us to experience. The action is not the goal, but the feeling the action brings is. We seek money for the necessities and pleasures that it provides that make us happy. We seek entertainment to feel happy. We participate in various activities for the joy we feel in doing them. We get good at sports for the freedom from having to think that being "in the zone" allows. We read to get lost in the thoughts of others, which again entertains or informs, taking us to feelings of happiness or contentment. We perform certain actions out of a sense of duty, which allows us to feel contented about doing the right thing.

As we can see, there is a common set of feelings at the goal of all of our actions. The actions that we perform that cannot be tied directly, at its root to feelings of peace, contentment, joy and happiness are few indeed. If we understand that all we do is really not for the doing, but for the emotional experience behind it, then we might ask ourselves, "Why am I focusing on the cause, when I could focus on the desired effect instead?"

If we really saw the ultimate goal behind everything we do is to feel some type of positive feeling, we just might begin to understand the importance that feeling good actually holds in our lives. If we understood this importance, maybe, just maybe, we might start to adjust our priorities or values to better reflect the attainment of what is most important in our lives.

If we know we want to be happy, and if we see that we do ten different things every day that all, at their root, point to wanting to experience happiness, then we might be able to do the things we do in a way that helps us experience our real goal sooner. Or we might see that some of the things we do get in the way of the ultimate feeling we are seeking. Maybe we don't need what amounts to a fancy, time consuming trigger anymore but can trigger ourselves directly to the feeling. Once we see how to trigger a feeling automatically, maybe we can decide to feel how we want to feel without the need of triggers, or with easy ones we set up for ourselves instead. We can begin to prioritize the feelings we treasure over the actions that we mistakenly thought we valued.

This doesn't mean we stop doing; it does mean we do what really is important knowing why we are really doing it, and it also means that we spend more time in the final state of mind that an experience is being done to achieve.

Our attachment to the triggers is very high, but if we try and see how we are actually able to feel the root emotions we crave on demand, we loosen the grip of many less-than-useful entertainments we currently hold dear. When we start living our lives mindful of why we do what we do, and with less intrusion of thought, then we lessen the need to live life through the activities of others. We pull life back into ourselves instead of living for what is outside of our states of mind.

Prioritizing happiness means behaving in a way where we trigger happiness for its own sake, whenever we choose to do so during the day. It means staying in a state of contentment throughout our day. It means not allowing the other states of mind that others who interact with us have pull us away from our most valued states. It means not valuing a belief or a supposed need over the peace and joy inherent within. Ultimately it means letting go of the learned adult who needs complicated triggers to feel good, and instead returning to the viewpoint of the young child, who knows they enjoy being happy, and that they can be happy doing whatever they are doing.

When we prioritize our state of mind as most important, we can approach any circumstance and ask ourselves, "What is it that I ultimately want out of this?" When we can see the endpoint before we start, we make it that much easier to get there faster.

If we ask ourselves this question before we start each day, we instantly begin to align ourselves and our actions with feeling good throughout the day. Each time we have a choice to perform an action or even think a thought that will take us out of the states of mind that we value most highly, we can instead remember our priorities, and decide not to stray.

The driver next to us shares a view of their finger. We can choose to join them in an angry state, or we can choose to stay in a happy or peaceful space instead. Do we value being angry or being happy? Which feeling would we choose to experience if we calmly stepped out of the situation and remembered we had the choice?

Now we realize we do have the choice, in every moment of our lives, and we can make better choices.

EXERCISE 5: THE CLASSROOM OF LIFE

When we are in school, we are in an artificial simulation of life. We are told things, we are shown how things work, and we are taught about various events, actions and beliefs. It is an artificial microcosm of the real school: life. When we finish school, the learning doesn't end. The lessons are always there, the opportunities to better understand and experience life always surround us, when we see that life is really a school.

Since life isn't organized quite like the schools we grew up attending, we need to add familiar elements into our lives to return ourselves to understanding that we go out into the world everyday to learn and to take tests. When we see this, we can better use the school of life, as it was really meant to be used.

As with school, life has a lesson it wants to teach. The simple subject for life's lessons is ultimately this: prioritize your state of mind, and stay in your prioritized state whenever you choose. Life throws little tests at us all day, seeing if we really value our positive state. It gives us opportunities and reminders all day long to push us away from what we value, or to pull us to deeper connections with our inner joy.

So when you wake up, align yourself with your highest priority. State it to yourself upon awakening. You can state, "I choose to be happy today," or "Today, I will be peace." Decide what your highest priority will be and state it aloud to yourself. Repeat it to yourself until it is ingrained and you believe it. Then make a point to remind yourself once an hour of this priority again. Repeat ingraining this decision as necessary throughout your day. Reinforce it with a smile, or by closing your eyes and connecting with your inner joy for a few moments.

Remember these feelings are why we do what we do. Then watch how the classroom that is life tests us during the day, trying to distract us from this feeling. Watch how the traffic doesn't move quite as we would like it to. Instead of shaving an extra minute or two it adds three to our morning commute. Or watch how that traffic light seemed to know you were coming, and changes just in time to catch you.

Little things will appear to tempt us away from our happiness all day long. We have to remember that the traffic light's color is not more important than our happiness, nor is a tick or two on the clock a determinate of how happy we can be.

Interacting with your classmates (your co-workers!) will produce numerous opportunities to practice steadfastness to your priority. Some may inadvertently do or say something to try to draw you away, while others may appear to make it their mission to take you out of your state. Don't let any of them succeed! In these moments remind yourself, this little perceived slight, or rudeness is coming from someone who has yet to connect with their childlike joy. Or know that words can be easily misunderstood. Understand it wasn't really meant to pull you down but is just the nature of unclear personal expression and incomplete interaction.

By staying clearly connected to your own center of joy, you not only feel better, you help the other to see that there is another way. Your inner joy reminds them of their own space of peace within and can help them to think of changing their priorities as well. The best teacher is your action, and when others see you smiling through adversity, it can encourage them to strive to do the same. When you watch yourself smiling in a challenging moment, you can pat yourself on the back because life threw you a little pop quiz, and you passed!

It doesn't hurt to have reminders around you during your day to help you establish happiness as your daily priority. As with anything else you learn, practice helps to perfect any lesson, and remembering to practice this lesson is key. Write simple sticky notes like "Prioritize Happiness", or the shorthand "PH". Use one that says, "Remember to Be Happy" or "RTBH" and put them wherever you spend a lot of time. You can also use computer sticky notes or wear a bracelet or necklace reminder. Anything that will quickly and easily make you remember your real priority over and over during your day will help to instill this new conscious remembrance of your priority into your daily life.

When you arrive home in the evening, class is not over. The deepest lessons are actually now in session. Interacting with your loved ones is where all of your practice must come to its highest focus. Stay attuned to your joy when your spouse yells at you for doing something they've labeled stupid. When they give you the silent treatment for forgetting to do what they wanted, stay with your joy. When your child spills milk, stay focused. Continue to remember your joy.

When your child hugs you goodnight, feel their love and stay with your inner joy. When your spouse forgives you, feel their love and stay in your inner joy. It is good to appreciate the love you experience at home, and to simultaneously keep connected to your inner joy. That way you don't become dependent on whether the outer love is coming to you or not, but you stay connected with your inner, unlimited, always-available source of happiness. Praise and blame, love and hate will come and go, but your inner peace will always be there.

Just before you go to sleep, again align yourself with your inner bliss, breathing into it and letting it flow through you. Allow your connection to continue into your sleep and you will find your dreams can also be permeated with experiencing your new priority. You will sleep better and more easily, and you will awaken refreshed and excited for another day in the classroom of life where the main course of instruction is Staying Connected to Your Inner Peace 101!

11) GRATITUDE

Gratitude is simply the act of being thankful. It can be directed towards life, or to a power greater than ourselves, or to the essence, source and creator of all. It is the single most important generator of happiness. When we connect to it, we are acknowledging that things could be different, things could be worse, and we are happy that things are the way they are. When we are grateful, we are also acknowledging that we are not approaching life as an entitlement, but as a gift. All the bountiful things we experience could be gone, but they're not, and we're happy to be able to experience them.

Thankfulness can be used as a trigger to our inner joy whenever we choose. There are hundreds or thousands of little things to be grateful for in our lives every single day, if only we could again look at life through the eyes of a young child and stop taking the moments of life for granted.

As a child, everything was new and amazing. The kitchen drawer holding all the plastic containers meant hours of joyful exploration for your toddler-self. Each new container was another treasure just awaiting to be examined, picked up with these wonderful fingers, held and felt, then tossed unceremoniously onto the floor as it was now time for the next container's examination. Crawling or haltingly taking a step or two was an experience to rejoice in as now the world was within reach. Mobility that we take for granted now, held such promise of delight for us when we were young children.

If we see life through the eyes of a child, there are even more things to be grateful for. Opportunities for gratitude are in abundance through the eyes of our young ones. A present at Christmas, wrapped in red and green paper is a source of delight for a one-year-old. This wonderful, crinkly paper is the best gift ever. Watching how it moves and flexes when you hold it is prime entertainment. Seeing what it does when you throw it is pure delight. Watching how it tears, hearing the sound the tearing makes, feeling the ripping paper in little hands- wow! And then mommy says, "Open it." What does that even mean? This new red and green toy is fascinating! Mommy rips the paper and tosses it aside. Crawling to retrieve it - why would she treat a new toy with such disregard!

A box of tissues is hours of fun waiting to happen. A little ball can be all a child needs for more hours of joy. Learning to crawl opens up a world of exploration. The first steps are incredible achievements promising an even wider circle of influence and exploration.

Life is ever new and ready to enjoy when we do not take anything for granted, but instead recognize opportunities for gratitude.

We hop in the car now and find ourselves miles away in minutes. What would have been a day's journey a couple of hundred years ago turns into a half hour drive listening to our favorite tunes or youtube channel to allay the monotony. Opportunity for gratitude. We eat lunch in a fancy restaurant built on ground where our ancestors may have hunted game a few centuries earlier. Opportunity for gratitude.

We vote in an election and look around the room and see, others who may not be as rich, or not the right sex, or not the right color to have been allowed to do this very act a couple of hundred years earlier. Opportunity for gratitude.

Yes, the world we live in has so much to be grateful for. The time we live in has so much that it didn't hold for those who lived before us. We are alive in a time full of change, and we are lucky enough to be able to have the perspective of seeing how things were before and after great advances like the cell phone or the internet.

Our business lives are full of amazing advances to be grateful for as well. The opportunity to interact with people throughout the world on a daily basis is another example of how broad life has become for us, and it is another thing to not take for granted. We can click a page on a screen and see what happened at any place in the world this day. We can watch what is happening live in various locations around the globe. We can date and even marry people from anywhere. Life has so many opportunities for us to explore. Today we can have numerous experiences our great-grandparents couldn't even dream of.

When we begin to see our lives through these lenses of perspective, we can see that we have so much to be grateful for, much of which we usually forget. Other basics that we take for granted when we have them are health, sanity, our functioning senses, freedom, sunlight… the list goes on and on. So, pick something, or a lot of things that resonate with you, and be grateful.

Feel how being grateful feels in your body. Notice how you feel happy, how contentment arises. Realize that when you are grateful you are aligning with your inner joy. You aren't fighting against what is, but are acknowledging what is, and celebrating it. Doing this puts us in the flow of our inner joy and helps us stay there.

As a young child there were moments of discord, but the large majority of our time was spent being grateful for the things we had. We celebrated them with the sheer enjoyment we gave them and with the total attention we put on them. We didn't think about life, we lived it. We accepted things the way they were and enjoyed them as they were. This simple, child-like expression points to the essence of gratitude: appreciating what is. The more we do this, the happier we will find our life experience.

Happiness cannot exist without acceptance of this moment. When we are fighting against this moment, the prime lawyer demanding change is the mind. It presents a case, it discusses its options, then it usually does nothing about the situation, other than complain and keep us from finding the joy in the situation instead. Flowers don't complain about the sun being on the other side of the field every morning. They turn their faces to experience it, then follow it all day, accepting that this is the way things are.

When we accept our lives as they are, we bring a lightness to everything we experience, and if things need to change, we are able to approach them from a more creative state of mind. Would you rather make a decision about your future when you are angry, or when you are happy? Are you more fully able to access your inner resources when you are angry, or when you are happy?

Everything works better and flows more smoothly when we are in positive, happy states of mind. Anger and other emotions that shade happiness have their small, limited uses, and should be applied sparingly and consciously, then put down. Living from happiness and other positive emotions aligns us with the flow of life and most consistently take us to a life we can celebrate living.

12) ALLOWING OURSELVES TO BE HAPPY

Watch how life changes when you are happy more often. See how decisions change, how your perspective on daily events improves, how your overall need to find activities to make you happy decreases when everything makes you happy. Notice how your interactions with people change, and how you approach all the tasks of your life.

Give yourself permission to be happy *now*. Why wait for an exterior event, only to find that it didn't do the trick, or that it was just another temporary fix for a permanent issue. When we put some great event out ahead of us and say, "When such and such happens, then I'll be happy," we are setting ourselves up to fail. The event that seemed so huge when we first envisioned it, the hilltop in the distance, becomes the next step on our journey of life when we arrive there. It isn't such a big deal when you are at the step before it, although when you are miles away it seems like a huge accomplishment. When you set up some event in the distance as your happiness trigger, you will always need some big event in the far future as your trigger. You will never be reach it. Your vision will always be a hundred steps ahead, and you will never allow yourself to take joy in the current step as it is so mundane in comparison to that lofty one way ahead.

Learn to appreciate the current step. Celebrate where you are now! Be happy in this very moment, for this very moment. Don't wait until some imagined perfect time to be happy. Setting up this story is training yourself to never be happy. Change that foolish pattern today!

There are at least two ways to see every event in life. When you know one way empowers you more than the other, why choose the less empowering one? Allow yourself to grab your power today, right now! Don't put it off any longer! That perfect day with all of the perfect circumstances is nothing more than a fantasy in the mind. It doesn't exist in real life anymore than most of the other thoughts the mind entertains on a daily basis. Don't fall into that trap anymore. When we live in today, we can allow ourselves to be happy in this day. And not later in the day, not when we get home at night, not when we are cuddled up with our loved one in bed. Right now. At this moment as we are commuting to work. Happiness should start at the beginning of the day and continue throughout the day.

Happiness becomes a habit when we practice it all day every day. As one of the most important habits to cultivate, we must learn to allow it to happen. This means accepting that we are worthy enough to be happy now. Realize that there is no standard of achievement that, once reached, will allow us to be happy. We have all that we need to be happy right now. What we are now is it! We didn't need a set of accomplishments as a one year old to be happy, and we don't need them now as an adult. Give yourself permission, right now, to be happy again!

The more we tend to set up hurdles against allowing happiness, the more distance we put between ourselves and our birthright of experiencing our inner joy. It is artificial for us to believe we can only be happy after A, B and C happen. How can we be happy then, when we will certainly set up new barriers D, E, and F in order to be happy?

Some of us think we need to withhold allowing happiness in order to drive us to reach our goals. We believe that if we are happy now, we will not have the drive necessary to achieve. The truth is that if we are involved in a goal that precludes being happy, we should probably reexamine the worthiness of the goal. If the goal is more important than being happy, we must ask is it something we really want, or is it just a distraction from our true ultimate goal? Most times we also need to look deep enough to realize the true goal of the goal is a positive feeling, and if we are missing out on the positive feeling now, delaying it for later, is this really the best way to reach that true goal?

When we are marching down a path of our own choosing, we are better able to make the journey when we allow ourselves to enjoy each step we take. Most times we find it is not the goal anyway, but the journey we take to make it there that is the most important experience. We grow most by walking along the path, not by reaching its end. When we are joyous along the path, we are able to spend most of our time growing in a state that maximizes our growth potential.

Experiments with plants show they grow fastest in positive atmospheres and humans thrive under these same conditions. When we feel joyful and surround ourselves with positive thoughts, people and circumstances, we can grow more, achieve more and appreciate life more. Why would we choose to have less for even one more day?

Now that we are no longer ignorant of what is real and what is imagined in the world of the mind, we can allow ourselves to choose feelings that are best for us, states of mind which connect us to that same place we let go of as a young child.

As children we trusted our parents and their society. We let go of inner joy which we held dear so that we could better fit in and gain their love and accolades. Now we see they didn't know any better, just as we didn't, until now. In this moment, we can forgive them and ourselves, and accept that life has a higher meaning than we formerly knew.

Now we know life is about staying in touch with our core of joy, and we have many tools to do so. We can appreciate and even be thankful for this new knowledge and express our thankfulness by experiencing it every day and by sharing it with the world as much as we can. As we share, we discontinue our selfish hoarding of our greatest gift to the world and begin giving the best we have to give to all.

13) HEALTHY BODY, USEFUL CHEMICALS

A quick note: I'm not a doctor, and nothing in this chapter is medical advice. These are general wellness ideas. For anything specific to your health — and before changing your diet, your exercise, or any medication — please talk with a qualified professional.

No book on happiness could be complete without a recognition of the need to have a healthy body. When we are sick, we have a very difficult time even thinking of being happy. When we are having deeper health issues, happiness can sometimes vanish from our horizon. Ironically these are the times when we need happiness the most, but we have the hardest time connecting to it.

The healing powers of joy and laughter are well documented. As with decisions in life, when it comes to our health, it is the same. Happiness promotes better decisions and it supports healthier lives. More happiness translates into less stress. More happiness allows the body to produce chemicals that support a stronger, more vibrant existence. Connecting to your inner joy is like giving yourself a boost of the most potent vitamins every day. Remembering happiness each day, keeps the doctor away!

Of course, we need to eat right. This means making sure the diet includes a large amount of living foods – fruits and vegetables. We should always eat in moderation and keep a balanced diet. We need to listen to our bodies and eat what the body needs, not necessarily what the taste buds want. We should eat when we are hungry, not necessarily when it is time to eat. We should stop eating a few hours before sleeping so that the digestion process is well along before we go to sleep. Our diet should keep us at a weight that helps us feel energized, not slothful.

Drinking water is an underrated necessity in a healthy lifestyle. Drinking fresh, clean water helps keep everything in the body flowing. Our bodies are mainly water, so we need to replenish the repository daily. A little juice from fruits is ok, but water by itself is what the body needs to thrive. Target the medically recommended amount for your size, and moderate this amount based on listening to your body. Bodies communicate their needs, if only we can listen. Whether it is dry eyes, or dry skin, or even a headache, the body has ways of telling us it is thirsty. We need to listen and give it what it needs.

We also must be sure to exercise every day, whether it be aerobics, or just walking. We need to take care of the heart and the muscles so that they will always serve us well. The heart is the most critical muscle, and it needs to be exercised daily. This means twenty minutes a day minimum of aerobic exercise. What qualifies as aerobic differs for all of us. For some who are not in great shape walking can raise the heartbeat to an aerobic level. For others a brisk walk or jog will do the trick. Dancing can be aerobic. The key is finding an enjoyable activity and doing it consistently.

 Our bodies need the stimulus of movement to keep us healthy and to connect us to happiness, just as they needed as children. As a young child, we had energy in amazing abundance. We were always moving, jumping, getting into one thing after another. When you are healthy and connected to your inner joy, this child-like energy is a natural occurrence.

Energy, movement and joy go hand in hand in hand. When we are missing one, the others can bring it back, or they can all disappear. When we feel lethargic, we have none of these three. This is the time to start moving. Movement will bring more energy, and with more energy comes a higher possibility to connect to positive emotional states. Or start to feel good. Trigger happiness inside and connect with your inner joy. When you are happier, you will find yourself with more energy and a higher will to move. Movement and energy feed on one another, helping grow all three. The same recipe holds true when we find ourselves in a negative emotional state. Start moving and let the other two grow, or smile, and connect with the will to start the other two.

Movement, energy, and joy are like the three sides of a triangular pill we must feed ourselves every day. When we do, the quality of life we experience is increased. Making their presence a habit is key in helping us to transform our lives.

Assuring we stay balanced in our activities is an important habit to cultivate. Everything in our world goes through cycles, and we are no exception. We must alternate between waking and sleep, being sure to get the amount of sleep our bodies need, not stuffing, or starving the body. Too much sleep can make the body lethargic, and too little sleep can make the mind fuzzy. We need periods of high energy, followed by periods of rest. Keeping these opposites balanced will give us the feeling of living a balanced life. The work time should always be balanced by the down time. The vacation is as important as the work. We should shape our weekends to be as rejuvenating as we need them to be.

We must engage in activities that recharge us. In order to accomplish this, it is good to understand the type of person we are. Do we enjoy being in groups of people? If we are energized by being with friends, we should make sure we spend enough time with them. If we are energized by spending quality time with ourselves, then we need to assure that this activity has its time. We are all different in what inputs give us energy, and which ones sap us of energy, but when we are able to connect to our joy in any situation, we are better able to be energized no matter what the circumstance.

When we keep our bodies healthy, happy, energized, and balanced, we allow our bodies to produce chemicals that support the continuation of these important habits. Just as muscles and bones support the frame of our bodies, the body's hormones or chemicals support our emotional and energetic lives. Without an even, healthy secretion of chemicals, the body is soon pretty useless to anyone. When we have an imbalance, all sorts of maladies arise. We eat well and exercise to help the body have a good flow of nutrients, oxygen and fluids, so that it has everything it needs to produce the chemicals necessary for a healthy experience in the body.

Our bodies are like a wonderful recipe for pancakes. All the right ingredients must be added together at the right time and in the right quantities, and then mixed to just the right consistency, then cooked at the right temperature for just the right amount of time in order to achieve great pancakes. Our bodies demand the same precision from their many parts in order to produce the chemical mix we need to thrive. We can't just ingest one drug (or chemical, like caffeine) and expect it to have the power to make everything alright. We should understand that it is actually much more likely to throw the whole finely-tuned machine out of balance than it is to help it achieve higher levels of operation. A healthy body, energized with movement, in tune with its inner joy will combine to produce more of the same when these three ingredients are mixed in the correct proportions on a daily basis. Forget the butter, and the pancakes just aren't right; forget the movement, and the joy doesn't have the same solid support.

The human machine is an extremely complicated set of interactions, and we must respect that it needs more maintenance than the fanciest of cars. In order to keep everything humming smoothly, we must eat right to give it the nutrients it needs to produce the correct chemical balance for a particular body. We must drink water to allow it to keep everything flowing, from the good nutrients around the body to the unnecessary waste products out of the body. We must listen to it and follow its needs. We should keep it clean, promote healthy teeth and healthy, chemical free skin. Our skin absorbs more than we tend to think. We should understand that the things we put on our skin can get inside our bodies, so be sure the things we feed our skin are useful for our bodies.

The newest part of the body that science now recognizes as a key helper is the community of microorganisms, collectively known as the microbiome. First, we need to recognize that this exists, and it is a critical part of our healthy functioning bodies. Therefore, we must tend to it as something we want to have thrive and stay in a good balance. When we eat live, healthy foods, we are feeding the biome too. A balanced biome assists the body in maintaining a good mood, and an imbalanced biome is a contributor to bad moods and ill health.

When we allow our mouths and hands to have a certain healthy balance of microbes (as icky as that may sound!) then we are giving our bodies what they need. This is part of why many health experts now caution against over-relying on antibacterial soaps and harsh sanitizers. Would we knowingly use something that would kill our liver (oops, many of us do – liquor)? Or our lungs (oops again, many of us do with the smoke we inhale). It is also worth being thoughtful with antibiotics. They are powerful and genuinely important when a doctor prescribes them — and, like anything powerful, they work best used exactly as directed, rather than reached for at the first sign of trouble. (Always follow your doctor's guidance.)

EXERCISE 6: HEALTHY LIVING

Examine your daily routine and see where you are using chemicals that do not promote health. Cut back on substances that tend to disrupt your natural energy and mood, like excess caffeine and energy drinks. Add more fruit and vegetables to your daily diet. Eat at least two fruits a day and two or three helpings of vegetables or nuts every day. Drink 50 to 65 ounces of water every day. Reduce then eliminate the junk food that adds no positive nutrients to your body. Exercise at least 30 minutes a day. Either walk or jog or run, depending on your level of fitness, or dance. Smile and laugh more during your day. Add these like good medicines and take your daily dose of each happily and in good measure.

14) LOVE

Sharing happiness is as important as nurturing it within. Yes, we must first recognize and grow it inside, then we must cultivate enough to share it with others. When we share our happiness, we are expressing our love for all. We are also saying we love ourselves and are confident enough to share this self-love with the world.

The world in turn will reflect the love we share back to us. It is very difficult for someone to reject another's smile. When someone smiles at us, we usually return it in kind. When we smile at people every day, we soon get a reputation for being a cheerful person, and we light up every room we enter. People always feel happier around happy people, so when we become that happy person, we find ourselves surrounded with positive feedback on our mood.

We share love by behaving in a manner that is congruent with our happiness. We love ourselves, and we demonstrate this love by giving ourselves the highest emotions every day. The fact that this is a priority in our lives shows that we have high self-esteem. How else could we feel happy when others don't necessarily share this feeling, and how else would we have the confidence to share this happiness outwardly with others if we didn't feel confidence inside?

We give love to others when we treat them kindly. We smile, we listen, we share our time, and we freely give our compliments and our joy. Once this way of being becomes a part of our lives, we start to recognize that our happiness is not limited to us but can be a circle expanding far beyond us. We touch others with our love who touch others who touch others still.

We begin to learn that our happiness doesn't come in a finite measure. We have as much as we want to share every day. When we want to share two scoops, we have two scoops; when we want to share ten thousand helpings, we have ten thousand to share. Very quickly we realize that it is best to share more since when we share more, more flows through us!

Our closest relationships, those with our friends and family, give us the opportunity to expand even more our expression of love and caring. Many times, we take these relationships for granted and do not nurture them as we should. When we interact with those we care about the most, oftentimes we believe these are the people who should see "the real me." This usually means they see the good and the bad, the highs and the lows, and should especially be willing to deal with the lows. After all, she is my best friend, or he is my husband, right? The people we love the most sometimes will get the worst of us.

This changes when we become more tuned to our inner happiness. When we learn that happiness is our natural state, suddenly we realize that when we are out of sorts, it is not as natural an occurrence as we previously thought. It is a learned pattern that can be unlearned. It is caused by a blockage that isn't allowing the inner joy to flow freely. It isn't something that those most intimate with us must learn to deal with or to help us through. It's something telling us to be more aware and recognize what's stopping the flow of joy. Applying this solution instead of dumping on our loved ones improves our relationships immediately. It also improves our flow because we now employ a better way to get out of a funk.

Sharing happiness with our family and friends means being attentive to their needs. It means listening and truly being with them. It means spending quality time with them, interacting, communicating, and enjoying one another. When we do this, we find all of our relationships become deeper, and we also find that we now know how to take this new way of being out to the rest of the world. We take a genuine interest in the lives and concerns of others and lend an empathetic ear and smiling heart more easily than ever before.

Our need to criticize is reduced, and instead we compliment more. The carrot can be shared by all, and the stick can be thrown away. How much better will our relationships be when instead of assuming low or bad intentions drive the actions of others, we can instead know that others actually only are driven by good intentions, even if sometimes only seen from a limited perspective? The mind thinks it is adding value by finding faults, when it is actually just creating a negative-facing worldview. When instead we add value by simply being happy, our whole world takes on a lightness and brightness that makes living a joy.

When happiness is our priority, caring is a natural outgrowth of feeling good more often. Sharing happens naturally as there is more good in us to do so. As a small child, sharing was natural; only as we grew did we have to be retaught that it was a good thing to do. Behaving in this manner provides positive feedback to our connection to our inner happiness. Feeling good and sharing it makes us feel even better and want to share it even more, so we create a win-win loop for our priority.

One amazing added benefit to this sharing is that over time, with this new perspective on life, we surround ourselves with other happy people, who also support our staying inside happiness. Some of the people are new people who also prioritize happiness, many are our friends and loved ones who, through our power of being happy, are now regularly happier themselves. Before long, through the power of prioritizing and sharing joy and love, we will find ourselves in a community of happy people all practicing the power of being happy.

15) KNOWING THIS, WHY AREN'T WE ALWAYS HAPPY?

Happiness is our birthright. The society we live in may grant us liberty and freedom, but the essence of who we are grants us happiness. Since happiness is such a basic part of who we are, feeling it and expressing is nothing but natural. When we feel strange when we find ourselves expressing happiness for seemingly no reason, we are listening to what we believe are the strictures of society and not our hearts.

We must leave this belief and understand that we have the right and the duty to express who we are at our essence. In fact when we don't, we create a society that sublimates feeling good and puts a multitude of activities that must be done between the happiness we yearn for and our current state of mind. This society says we need to do this before we can be happy, we need to accomplish that, participate in this, be that, and then we can be happy.

The truth is we can be happy because at our core we *are* happiness. That is why you crave this feeling and participate in all of these activities in the first place. Experiencing happiness is coming home to who you really are.

Much like a room can be dark only when there is no light, we can be angry only when we are not connecting with our inner happiness. We have light inside, and we can experience the lack of light. We do not have darkness inside unless we are hiding the light.

If happiness is our natural inner state, why aren't we always able to be happy? With the twenty, thirty, forty or more years of teachings we receive from society saying live life disconnected from our happiness, reinforced daily by those around us, it is a testament to the power of happiness that we still yearn to experience it at all.

Like a light that is hidden under a large pile of dirt, with more being piled on every day, we need to learn to consistently move the light, or remove the dirt. The dirt in our lives is what we hear and see from society and the expectations we have learned about the right way to behave. It is the need we have been taught to have to associate being happy with an event or experience. It is also the misunderstanding we have been made to believe that we are not really happiness at all, but the trappings of our life that obscure our happiness. We are taught we are the pile of dirt and not the light underneath, and we are given more dirt every day to add to that pile of who society would have us believe we truly are.

When we are being taught daily to obscure our truth, we must be diligent daily to clear the dirt, move our light, and stay aware of our true core. Every day, many times a day, we must consciously connect with our source. We must remember to be happy, tossing the dust that a day in any society will try to cover us with. We need to realize that society's game is "cover the light" and our game of "experience our inner light" must be played even harder in order to win every day.

Those around us in our work and even in our personal lives unwittingly play the opponent when they are not connecting with their inner light. When they parrot the teachings they learned, they are taking some of the dirt from their piles to give to your pile. We must stop letting this happen, and instead remove ourselves from this game.

The teachings of society are like a virus, and expressing happiness is our immune system. The more happiness we experience, the stronger our defenses become. We can't just be happy once and expect to win the game. It is an ongoing, daily, hourly viral infection society is unleashing against us, and we must be continuous in staying true to connecting to and expressing joy in our lives in the moments of our day. The sooner we understand that the very nature of our society is directly opposed to our own inner nature, the sooner we can see that it is the nature of this interaction to forget and need to be reminded again and again until we have played the game well enough and consistently enough to begin to build a community with values that are in tune with our nature.

When we stop needing anything to be happy, but just are happy, we begin to raise our self-esteem. When we express who we are through happiness, we stop pretending to be something we are not. Instead of listening to the teachings of society, we listen to the truth in our hearts. When we follow the truth in our hearts, we align with nature, and experience how easy and natural it becomes to be happy every day.

16) DAILY SELF-TALK: SUPPORTING HAPPINESS, OR UNDERMINING IT?

As a young child, there is no self-talk because there are no words yet. As we get older, we learn a language and begin the odyssey of living in self-talk. At first, we hear the voice and enjoy the novelty of words appearing in our heads. The words reflect a happy state and a child-like belief in positive things happening. The voice has use and we believe it. When things don't go our way, the voice supports us in feeling badly, and encouraging us to whine and cry. As we grow up and learn how not to be happy, the voice plays a large role in helping us to believe this is the right way to live. It does this by seeing things in a dimmer light, and by looking for things to criticize instead of to enjoy. It begins to see the half-empty glass in more and more things.

Now the voice is an integrated part of our lives. This means every day we get to listen to an opinion on everything we see and hear. It means becoming so used to this inner conversation that we take for granted that the voice is us thinking. The voice in our heads is many times more critical than approving. It looks for fault instead of beauty. It colors our view of life in a somewhat cynical shading instead of a hopeful joyousness.

The self-talk of criticism is extremely destructive. Entertaining a conversation in our heads where we cut another person down is not worthy of the energy we use to form the thoughts. We believe it is natural to occasionally think ill towards another, but if we really look at what we are doing when we do this, we can see that we are not really in control but are just allowing the basest beliefs in the mind to run free. It is just as bad when we direct this flow of negative feelings towards ourselves. Again, this is a poor use of our mental energy, and does no good towards making our highest priority a reality.

If we could have the perspective of looking back on any self-talk conversation like this, in a happier, more peaceful moment, we would not have allowed the self-talk to take place. So, we have to bring this better perspective into the moment the un-empowering self-talk is occurring instead of wishing we had done so later on.

The voice of self-talk is so much us that we never stop to believe otherwise. Not for a moment do any of us say, "Where did that thought come from?" or "I don't really believe that, do I?" To question the source of the voice would mean we are hearing voices, right, so we believe it is us talking, and that everything it says is true.

Now, what if we stopped believing that for a minute or two? What if instead we believed we could train this voice to see a better world? What if we could teach it to be quiet instead of always giving its opinion?

Taking control of the self-talk is one of the most important keys to returning to your child-like joy. We do this through the simple recognition that just because a thought is in our head doesn't necessarily make it true. It doesn't necessarily even make it a thought we believe. Our experience and conditioning create the mechanism that powers self-talk, and we can change these at will. We can listen or not, at will. Simple techniques like meditation help us to strengthen the muscle of inner silence.

With this new understanding, we can begin to see self-talk in a brand-new light. Like telling the emperor that he has no clothes, learning that we have dominion over self-talk changes everything. We can see we are not the victims of its whims anymore, but the masters of its direction. Shining a light on it allows us to see it is a tool for us to use as needed, and to let go of when it is not useful. Simple self-awareness will make sure that self-talk never has the power over us that it once had.

We can now use it to feel good when we want to and watch when it is making us feel badly and stop it from doing so. It has been on auto-pilot for most of our lives, so it will take diligence to help it to become our friend and helper again. We need to realize we receive big hints of when it is running awry through our feelings. When we feel down or negative, it is a great reminder to look at our self-talk and to adjust it so that we can feel better. Since joy is our inner nature, it takes self-talk to take us out of it, so when self-talk is full on criticizing ourselves or others, we feel out-of-joy, and we need to recognize the cause of this and correct it at once.

Changing negative self-talk to positive self-talk works wonders immediately. Feelings follow its direction almost instantaneously. Cutting it off also allows our real essence to flow again. We only need to remember we are the boss, not the words flowing through our heads. Self-talk only has the power we give it, so we need to give it the power to uplift our experience of life, not the opposite.

17) SUPPRESSING EMOTIONS: THE SPOCK MENTALITY

Many of us (so called left brainers!) grew up idolizing logic over emotion. The personification of this was Spock, the logical scientist who was able to subvert his emotional side. Even though he felt happiest when he let his emotions free, the overarching lesson we got from his story was the supremacy of controlling and never expressing emotion.

In real life it is actually stronger to show and share emotions, but this truth is sometimes lost on many of us. Living in a mechanized, sanitized society, we forget that it is good to be human, to act as human, and to let human emotions show in our daily lives. The dehumanization of the workplace makes it easy to believe emotions have no place, but this is not true.

When we show our inner happiness, we are acknowledging the truth about who we really are. We are having the strength to share our connection with our reality within. We are going against what we learned from school, from society, and from Spock when we assert the freedom to show our happiness when we are happy. We are being strong when we do not mind what others think about our sharing our happiness with the world.

So many people have been conditioned against sharing happiness that it takes an act of courage in certain instances to show this truth to the world. To change the world and make it a happier place for all takes a strength of character that believes it is right even in the face of many who may believe otherwise.

Logic doesn't die with the recognition of emotion but is actually bolstered by its expression. As with all other human acts, when we act logically while expressing our highest emotional states, we have the best results. Nothing is divorced from how we feel when we do it. Removing the extra added sensation of happiness from anything we do only lessens its effectiveness, so we should look to be happy, and to show our happiness whenever we can and wherever we can. The lessons we learned to the contrary need to be seen as faulty, and replaced with our new, deeper understanding of who we really are at the core.

18) THE HAPPINESS HABIT

As with anything important in our lives, we get better when we practice. The more we practice something, the more familiar we get with its nuances. The more we practice, the less we have to think about the details, as they become ingrained in us.

If we are learning to play an instrument like the flute, at first it is difficult to even hold it right. After days or weeks, we get comfortable holding it, but blowing across the mouthpiece doesn't feel natural. We practice more and holding it and making a sound come out becomes easier but putting our fingers on the right keys is hard. Eventually even this becomes rote, but only through hours and hours of practice. Many more hours of practice still are needed to become good at moving our fingers fast enough to make good music, and then we still must learn to connect what we see on a sheet of music with the movements of our hands and our breath. After years of diligent practice, the essentials of playing become habitual, and we have become a master of our instrument.

Relearning to connect to our happiness is no different. It takes daily practice to make connecting to happiness a habit. We must be diligent in our mission to be a person connected to inner joy. We must pick up the instrument of happiness daily and play it. We can't be afraid to miss notes either but know that this is a part of learning. If we make another person uncomfortable by being happy, it is not our duty to connect less with our inner truth, but only to accept this is part of the journey of creating a happier life and a happier world. Others will eventually connect to their inner happiness too, but it takes the pioneers to do it first in order to blaze the trail of acceptance for the others.

Everyday we must connect with our breath, go inside and feel that inner joy. We need to smile, we need to laugh, we need to stay in this joyous space when others try to share their less-than-joyous point of view with us. Practicing all of this each day will make it easier to do it a little better the next day. We can't expect to become masters of happiness overnight, but over time we will when we practice consistently.

When we make it habitual to smile, to breath and go within, to not follow our thoughts, but to live as life is happening, we become accustomed to the nuances of happiness, and we master our connection with and expression of our core bliss. We establish this habit by doing, again and again. It may be easy, or we may encounter obstacles, since society is built to move in the opposite direction, but whatever our experience, we will enjoy continuing to live in increasing mastery of happiness in all situations.

When we are sporadic in our practice, we aren't able to establish happiness as a habit in our lives. If we practice every now and then, we don't allow ourselves to experience happiness as a natural part of our lives.

When we learned to ride a bike, we had to practice in order to get good. After a little practice, we found that it was a lot of fun to continue practicing. Anytime we get really good at something, we have gone through to the point where practice is fun. We enjoy the doing, and we appreciate the results we experience.

Again, happiness is no different. When we are practicing being happy, we are happy. When we are connecting to our inner joy, we are joyous. This is a practice where we instantly experience the fruits of the practice.

Sometimes it helps to have reminders around you. A sticky note with the words "Happiness Habit," or the letters "HH" can be a reminder. A string around your wrist or finger can be a reminder. Even something as simple as a breath or a smile can serve as a reminder to help us connect to experiencing our core during our day. Enjoying the fruits of being happy will serve as incentive to keep us moving forward and deeper into the experience.

One day, after mastering practice, we will find that we have established the happiness habit. We are naturally in tune with being joyful without any effort. When we are in this state, we are continuously aware of our essence, and we can return to experiencing it in the blink of an eye. We know what we are and enjoy sharing it with the world. We know that we add value to the world by showing a happier way to be. We see more people around us living happier lives too. We know that we are now a positive influence in building a circle and a community of people who connect to their inner joy as a natural part of their daily lives.

19) THE POWER OF HAPPY: YOU ARE HAPPINESS

When we prioritize being happy, we are connecting to an aspect of our essence. To be joyful really is a pretty profound statement of knowing who we really are. We are not surly, angry, hurtful beings at our core, but instead we are happy, joyful, blissful, peaceful, and contented. To connect to and express this is to be in tune with the flow of our lives, and to experience the maximum energy of life.

To be in tune with this means we are experiencing the power of being happy. When we live each day consciously expressing the various emotions in the spectrum of happiness (bliss, joy, happiness, peace, contentment), we experience the power of happy. It means we see the world through better glasses, glasses more in tune with reality, and we experience the events of life through a truer perspective. The power of happiness lets us let go of blame and live in acceptance. We realize it is more important to be happy than to be right. It is more important to be at peace than to try to teach an unrequested lesson to another. It is better to enjoy our bubble of bliss than to live in someone else's gloomy imagined reality.

Staying connected with the power of happy means we value our state of being, and we nurture it daily. We share it with others and watch it grow for all. The power of happy acknowledges the ultimate reason we do almost anything we do, and it celebrates getting to the root of our needs instead of circling around but never diving in. When we are happy just because, we are diving into our essence and realizing we are happy and it is ok to show it. It is ok to laugh for no reason at all, or at something funny that just hits our minds. It is ok to express the happiness spectrum for the world to see because it is natural, and it is what we all want to experience. When we say it is ok to be happy by being happy, we give others that teaching too, and this is actually the only unrequested teaching really worth being taught, because at our essence, we are all yearning to learn it.

When we live in the power of happy, we are going back to the experience of life as a small child. We are enjoying living and enjoy the little things in life because we are paying attention to them instead of to thinking about and around them. When we are in the power of happy, we are truly alive again. We share with the world, not caring that others have not joined us yet, but instead knowing that this is what everyone needs, and when shared it will collectively create a better world for us all.

Ultimately, the practice of connecting with happiness, prioritizing happiness, and living in the power of happy shows us that at our core, we are nothing but the spectrum of happiness. We are bliss, we are joy, we are peace, contentment and happiness. This is the expression of our truest life. It is the feeling that we are in our essence. It is the best way we have to live our lives for ourselves and the world. When we live in the power of happy, we are living in the power of our essence, in the light that we are at our core.

The power of happy gives our lives a peace that we heretofore could not have imagined. It gives our dealings with others and our experience of ourselves a lightness and freshness that makes living new in every moment. The power of happy transforms our perspective on life and allows us to live as we were meant to live: in bliss.

A NOTE FROM THE AUTHOR

Thank you for spending this time with me — and with the joyful, blissful being you have always been underneath everything the world piled on top.

Everything in this book comes down to one quiet idea: you do not have to become happy. You already are happiness. The work was never to manufacture it, only to stop smothering it — and to let your natural joy come back to the surface, a little more each day. Be gentle with yourself as you practice. The four-year-old who couldn't stop smiling is still in there, and she has been waiting for you.

A Small Request

If this book helped you reconnect with your own joy, please consider leaving a short, honest review on Amazon, and sharing it with someone who could use a little more happiness in their life. Reviews are how a book like this finds the next person who needs it — even a few kind words make a real difference. Thank you for helping the happiness spread.

Continue the Journey

If you enjoyed this book, you may also like these, by G. Tyler Wright:

You Are Already It — A direct, simple guide to awakening, presence, and the reality of who you are.

How to Become Enlightened in 12 Days — A gentle, day-by-day path to presence and inner peace.

Three Easy Steps to Enlightenment — The essence, distilled into three small shifts in understanding.

I Do Not Exist and Neither Do You — A deeper look at the freedom beyond the separate self.

I Don't Care: The Reality of Who You Are — The blunt, liberating edge of the same truth.

The Stressed Mom's Reset — Reducing stress and reclaiming your peace, ten days to freedom.

You can find these and more at Transcendent-Writings.com.

About G. Tyler Wright

G. Tyler Wright writes about happiness, awareness, presence, and the realization of the joyful being we already are. His books point toward a single, freeing recognition: that peace and joy are not somewhere ahead of you to be earned, but your own nature, already here, waiting to be remembered.

the author.

9 781980 586395